THE MEDITERRANEAN MEAL PREP COOKBOOK

Discover vitality through the joy of Mediterranean dining. 'Feast Your Way to Vitality' invites you to savor delightful dishes, embrace well-being, and find happiness in a healthier you. Your journey to revitalization starts with every flavorful bite."

Frank C. Rivera

Table of content

Table of content

INTRODUCTION

Divulging the Mediterranean Mystery to Essentialness

In a world soaked with dietary patterns and prevailing fashions, the Mediterranean eating routine arises as a routine as well as a way of life, offering plenty of medical advantages that reach a long way past the plate. This dietary worldview, established in the sun-kissed districts encompassing the Mediterranean Ocean, has spellbound the consideration of well-being devotees and nutritionists the same for its comprehensive way to deal with prosperity.

Brief Outline of the Medical Advantages: Supporting the Body and Soul

The Mediterranean eating regimen remains a guide of well-being, eminent for its heart-accommodating characteristics and the possibility to fight off ongoing illnesses. Wealthy in olive oil, natural products, vegetables, entire grains, and lean proteins, this culinary custom has been connected to decreased dangers of cardiovascular issues and expanded life span. Besides, the consideration of omega-3 unsaturated fats from fish, combined with cell reinforcements from brilliant leafy foods, makes a wholesome cooperative energy that upholds mental capability and in general imperativeness.

Unique interaction: A Culinary Odyssey

Leaving on an individual excursion to embrace the Mediterranean eating routine, I found something beyond an approach to eating - I tracked down an association with culture, nature, and a significant feeling of prosperity. The smell of newly squeezed olive oil, the dynamic shades of ready tomatoes, and the strong kinds of spices and flavors turned into a necessary piece of my culinary story. This excursion isn't only about taking on an eating regimen; it's a festival of life, a combination of flavors that reverberate with the spirit.

Commitment of the Book: Divulging the Way to Essentialness

In "Enjoying Essentialness: A Mediterranean Culinary Undertaking," I welcome you to go along with me on an extraordinary experience toward a better and more dynamic way of life. This book rises above conventional cookbooks; it's a manual for injecting delight and comfort into your dinner prep schedule. Through cautiously arranged recipes, viable tips, and individual stories, you'll find the insider facts of Mediterranean cooking and open the possibility of reviving your well-being. Get ready to leave on a culinary excursion that supports your body as well as gives the pleasure of cooking and enjoying delectable, invigorating feasts into your routine.

Welcome to an existence where the craft of feast planning turns into a passage to imperativeness, and each nibble is a stage toward a better, more satisfied you. Allow the excursion to start.

Chapter 1: The Essence of Mediterranean Cuisine

Opening the Culinary Woven artwork

Welcome to the gastronomic excursion through the core of Mediterranean cooking, an enthralling embroidery woven with the best flavors, key fixings, and social importance. In this part, we dive into the actual substance of this culinary wonder, investigating the fortunes that make Mediterranean eating a fine art celebrated by foodies and culinary travelers the same.

Key Fixings and Their Medical Advantages

At the center of Mediterranean cooking lies an energetic cluster of fixings, each assuming a vital part in making an orchestra of flavors. Olive oil, with its brilliant tint, becomes the dominant focal point, as a cooking medium as well as an image of wellbeing. Wealthy in monounsaturated fats and cell reinforcements, it improves the flavor of dishes as well as adds to cardiovascular prosperity.

Tomatoes, sun-kissed and overflowing with pleasantness, are another key component. Loaded with lycopene, they offer an eruption of variety as well as a munitions stockpile of medical advantages, from elevating skin wellbeing to decreasing the gamble of specific tumors.

The Mediterranean table is embellished with an overflow of new leafy foods, from fresh cucumbers to delicious oranges, each bringing its exceptional arrangement of nutrients, minerals, and cell reinforcements. These fixings hoist the taste as well as add to the acclaimed life span related to Mediterranean eating regimens.

Social Bits of Knowledge and the Meaning of Mediterranean Feasting

Mediterranean cooking isn't just about the fixings; a social peculiarity mirrors the spirit of the district. From the Greek islands to the shores of Italy, each dish recounts a story, saturated with hundreds of years of custom. It's a festival of life, family, and the local area, where feasts are an outflow of affection and fellowship.

The meaning of the Mediterranean eating regimen goes past the plate. A way of life embraces effortlessness, balance, and the delight of relishing each chomp. The public part of eating is profoundly imbued, cultivating a feeling of association and shared encounters.

Appeal to Foodies and Culinary Travelers

For the insightful foodie, Mediterranean cooking is a gold mine ready to be investigated. Imagine yourself relishing the newness of a Greek serving of mixed greens, the zing of Spanish paella, or the deliciousness of Italian bruschetta. Each nibble is an identification of an alternate corner of the Mediterranean, a culinary experience that rises above geological limits.

The variety of flavors, the guileful utilization of spices and flavors, and the careful arrangement strategies appeal to the individuals who view food as food as well as an investigation of culture and craftsmanship.

All in all, Part 1 unwinds the enchantment of Mediterranean food, establishing the groundwork for a culinary campaign that goes past taste buds. It's an investigation of well-being, culture, and the sheer delight of enjoying the best flavors the Mediterranean brings to the table. Thus, lock in for an excursion through the sweet-smelling scenes and flavorful practices that make this cooking an overwhelming charm for food lovers around the world.

Chapter 2: Meal Prep 101 – Streamlining Your Cooking Routine

In the quick-moving world we live in, carving out opportunities for nutritious and home-prepared dinners can be a test. Part 2 plunges into the specialty of dinner prep, offering an exhaustive manual for smoothing out your cooking schedule. Whether you're a bustling proficient shuffling work responsibilities or part of a clamoring family, these tips are intended to make dinner arranging and planning a consistent piece of your way of life.

Productive Feast Making arrangements for Occupied Ways of life

Ace the Week after week Menu:

Make a week-after-week menu that lines up with your taste inclinations and nourishing objectives. This changes up your dinners as well as works on your shopping for food.

Clump Cooking Rudiments:

Embrace clump cooking to get ready bigger amounts of staples like grains, proteins, and sauces. This assists with timing during the week and guarantees you generally have a base to construct your feasts.

Shrewd Fixing Cross-over:

Pick recipes that share normal fixings to limit squandering and work on your basic food item list. This procedure additionally advances cost viability.

Taking care of Occupied Experts

Fast and Supplement Thick Recipes:

Find recipes that focus on effortlessness without settling on sustenance. Fast sautés, sheet dish meals, and one-pot ponders are phenomenal decisions for experts in a hurry.

Vital Prep Meetings:

Distribute explicit schedule openings during the week for dinner prep. This could be on the end of the week or an assigned weeknight, guaranteeing that you have arranged components prepared for fast gathering on more occupied days.

Put resources into Efficient Instruments:

Consider kitchen contraptions like a decent-quality blade, a food processor, or a sluggish cooker to facilitate the cooking system. These devices can be significant for time-lashed people.

Fledgling Agreeable Systems

Begin with Basic Recipes:

In the event that you're new to feast prep, start with simple and clear recipes. Bit by bit, as you gain certainty, you can explore different avenues regarding more complicated dishes.

Segment Control Methods:

Figure out how to successfully divide your feasts. Put resources into reusable holders to partition dinners into fitting servings, making it more straightforward to oversee divides and control calorie admission.

Fabricate a Collection of Go-To Recipes:

Distinguish a modest bunch of recipes that you appreciate and are not difficult to plan. Having a bunch of dependable go-to feasts diminishes choice weariness and works on your week-after-week arranging.

In rundown, Section 2 is your door to becoming the best at dinner prep. By embracing effective preparation, taking care of your particular way of life, and embracing novice amicable systems, you'll smooth out your cooking standard as well as partake in the advantages of better, custom-made dinners. Plan to change your kitchen into a space of culinary effectiveness and fulfillment.

Chapter 3: Quick and Wholesome Breakfasts

1. Mediterranean Avocado Toast

Portrayal: Begin your day with an explosion of energy! This avocado toast is roused by Mediterranean flavors, highlighting velvety avocado, cherry tomatoes, and a sprinkle of feta for a great curve.

Spending time in jail: 10 minutes

Cooking Style: No cooking required

Fixings:

2 cuts entire grain bread

1 ready avocado

1 cup cherry tomatoes, divided

2 tbsp feta cheddar, disintegrated

New basil leaves for decorating

Salt and pepper to taste

Guidelines:

Toast the entire grain bread cuts as you would prefer.

While toasting, pound the ready avocado in a bowl and season with salt and pepper.

Spread the squashed avocado uniformly over the toasted bread.

Top with split cherry tomatoes and disintegrated feta.

Embellish with new basil leaves.

Serve right away and relish the Mediterranean goodness!

2. Greek Yogurt Parfait with Blended Berries

Portrayal: A wellbeing cognizant and outwardly engaging breakfast! This Greek yogurt parfait consolidates the lavishness of yogurt with the pleasantness of blended berries, making it a delightful morning treat.

Spending time in jail: 5 minutes

Cooking Style: No cooking required

Fixings:

1 cup Greek yogurt

1/2 cup granola

1/2 cup blended berries (strawberries, blueberries, raspberries)

1 tbsp honey

Mint leaves for embellish

Directions:

In a glass or bowl, layer Greek yogurt at the base.

Add a layer of granola on top of the yogurt.

Disperse blended berries over the granola.

Shower honey over the berries.

Rehash the layers.

Embellish with mint leaves.

Partake in this healthy and protein-stuffed breakfast!

3. Spinach and Feta Breakfast Wrap

Depiction: A flavorful and fulfilling breakfast wrap loaded up with spinach, feta, and fried eggs. Loaded with supplements, it's ideally suited for a fast and supporting beginning to your day.

Spending time in jail: 15 minutes

Cooking Style: Burner

Fixings:

2 huge entire eggs, beaten

1 cup new spinach, cleaved

2 tbsp feta cheddar, disintegrated

1 entire wheat tortilla

Salt and pepper to taste

Olive oil for cooking

Directions:

In a dish, sauté hacked spinach in olive oil until shriveled.

Add beaten eggs to the container and scramble with spinach.

Season with salt and pepper.

Warm the entire wheat tortilla in a different container.

Place the fried egg and spinach combination on the tortilla.

Sprinkle disintegrated feta over the eggs.

Fold the tortilla into a wrap.

Serve quickly for a protein-pressed breakfast in a hurry!

4. Mediterranean Omelet Cups

Portrayal: These singular omelet cups are loaded up with Mediterranean goodness - tomatoes, olives, and feta. They're not difficult to make ahead for a fast and healthy breakfast.

Spending time in jail: 20 minutes

Cooking Style: Stove

Fixings:

4 huge eggs

1/4 cup cherry tomatoes, diced

2 tbsp Kalamata olives, hacked

2 tbsp feta cheddar, disintegrated

New oregano for embellish

Salt and pepper to taste

Guidelines:

Preheat the broiler to 350°F (180°C).

In a bowl, beat the eggs and season with salt and pepper.

Oil a biscuit tin and empty the beaten eggs equitably into each cup.

Appropriate diced tomatoes, hacked olives, and disintegrated feta among the cups.

Prepare for 15-18 minutes or until the eggs are set.

Decorate with new oregano.

Permit to cool somewhat before serving these tasty omelet cups.

5. Quinoa Breakfast Bowl with Products of the soil

Portrayal: A supplement stuffed breakfast bowl including quinoa, new organic products, and nuts. This healthy and fulfilling choice is great for those looking for well-being cognizant beginning of their day.

Spending time in jail: 15 minutes

Cooking Style: Burner

Fixings:

1/2 cup cooked quinoa

1/2 cup blended new organic products (berries, banana cuts)

2 tbsp nuts (almonds, pecans), slashed

1 tbsp honey

1/2 cup Greek yogurt

Directions:

Cook quinoa as per bundle directions.

In a bowl, layer cooked quinoa.

Add blended new products of the soil nuts on top.

Shower honey over the bowl.

Present with a spot of Greek yogurt.

Combine everything as one preceding partaking in this protein-rich breakfast bowl.

6. Mediterranean Egg Biscuits with Sun-Dried Tomatoes

Depiction: These exquisite egg biscuits are stacked with Mediterranean flavors, highlighting sun-dried tomatoes, feta, and spinach. They are ideal for a speedy and convenient breakfast, particularly for occupied people in a hurry.

Spending time in jail: 25 minutes

Cooking Style: Stove

Fixings:

6 huge eggs

1/2 cup sun-dried tomatoes, hacked

1 cup new spinach, finely hacked

1/4 cup feta cheddar, disintegrated

1/4 cup milk

Salt and pepper to taste

Guidelines:

Preheat the broiler to 375°F (190°C) and oil a biscuit tin.

In a bowl, whisk together eggs, milk, salt, and pepper.

Mix in hacked sun-dried tomatoes, spinach, and disintegrated feta.

Empty the blend equally into biscuit cups.

Prepare for 20-22 minutes or until the egg biscuits are set.

Permit them to cool somewhat before eliminating from the tin.

Partake in these tasty and protein-pressed egg biscuits for a delightful breakfast.

7. Tahini Banana Hotcakes

Depiction: A wind on exemplary hotcakes, these Tahini Banana Flapjacks carry a Mediterranean pizazz to your morning meal. The velvety tahini supplements the pleasantness of bananas for a great morning treat.

Spending time in jail: 15 minutes

Cooking Style: Burner

Fixings:

1 cup entire wheat flour

1 ready banana, crushed

1 cup milk

2 tbsp tahini

1 tbsp honey

1 tsp baking powder

Touch of salt

Cooking splash or margarine for the skillet

Directions:

In a bowl, whisk together flour, squashed banana, milk, tahini, honey, baking powder, and salt until very much consolidated.

Heat a container over medium intensity and coat with a cooking splash or spread.

Pour 1/4 cup of hitter onto the search for gold hotcake.

Cook until bubbles structure on a superficial level, then flip and cook the opposite side until brilliant brown.

Rehash until everything player is utilized.

Serve these Tahini Banana Hotcakes with a sprinkle of honey for a Mediterranean-motivated breakfast.

8. Shakshuka-Roused Breakfast Burrito

Portrayal: A good and tasty breakfast burrito motivated by the Center Eastern dish Shakshuka. Loaded up with flavored tomatoes, poached eggs, and feta, it's a healthy and fulfilling start to the day.

Spending time in jail: 20 minutes

Cooking Style: Burner

Fixings:

2 huge entire eggs

1/2 cup canned diced tomatoes

1/4 cup red chime pepper, diced

1/4 cup onion, diced

1 clove garlic, minced

1/2 tsp cumin

1/2 tsp paprika

Salt and pepper to taste

1 huge entire wheat tortilla

2 tbsp disintegrated feta

Directions:

In a dish, sauté diced onion and red ringer pepper until relaxed.

Add minced garlic, cumin, paprika, salt, and pepper. Cook for an extra moment.

Empty canned diced tomatoes into the container and stew until marginally thickened.

Make two wells in the tomato blend and break eggs into each well.

Cover the container and poach the eggs until cooked as you would prefer.

Warm the entire wheat tortilla and spoon the tomato and egg blend onto it.

Sprinkle disintegrated feta over the top.

Fold the tortilla into a burrito and partake in this Shakshuka-roused breakfast bend.

9. Mango and Pistachio Short-term Oats

Depiction: A flavorful and nutritious short-term oats recipe with the pleasantness of mango and the mash of pistachios. Set it up the prior night for a problem-free and fulfilling breakfast.

Spending time in jail: 10 minutes (in addition to expediting drenching)

Cooking Style: No cooking required

Fixings:

1/2 cup moved oats

1/2 cup milk (dairy or plant-based)

1/2 cup mango lumps

1 tbsp honey

1 tbsp pistachios, slashed

Guidelines:

In a container or bowl, join moved oats and milk.

Add mango lumps and honey, blending to blend well.

Cover and refrigerate for the time being.

In the first part of the day, give the oats a decent mix and top with cleaved pistachios.

Partake in these Mango and Pistachio Short-term Oats for a reviving and supplement-pressed breakfast.

10. Mediterranean Breakfast Quesadilla

Depiction: An exquisite and protein-rich quesadilla including Mediterranean fixings like hummus, cherry tomatoes, and spinach. This morning meal choice rushes to plan and is ideal for occupied mornings.

Spending time in jail: 15 minutes

Cooking Style: Burner

Fixings:

2 entire wheat tortillas

1/2 cup hummus

1 cup new spinach

1/2 cup cherry tomatoes, cut

1/4 cup feta cheddar, disintegrated

Olive oil for cooking

Directions:

Spread hummus uniformly on one side of every tortilla.

Place a tortilla, hummus side up, on a warmed skillet.

Layer new spinach, cut cherry tomatoes, and disintegrated feta on top.

Place the subsequent tortilla, hummus side down, on the fixings.

Cook until the base tortilla is brilliant brown, then flip and cook the opposite side.

When the two sides are cooked, eliminate from the skillet and let it cool somewhat.

Cut into wedges and partake in this Mediterranean Breakfast Quesadilla.

Stimulating Morning Recipes for Occupied People

Could it be said that you are a hard worker with a clamoring plan? Begin your day with an explosion of energy through these fast and nutritious morning recipes custom-fitted for occupied people.

Short-term Oats with Berries and Almonds:

Set up the prior night for an in-and-out breakfast.

Loaded with fiber and cell reinforcements from berries, and a protein help from almonds.

Avocado and Egg Breakfast Wrap:

A protein-stuffed breakfast that requires minutes to plan.

Avocado gives sound fats to support energy.

Greek Yogurt Parfait with Nuts and Honey:

High-protein Greek yogurt keeps you full and centered.

Nuts add crunch and solid fats, while honey gives normal pleasantness.

Green Smoothie Bowl:

Mix spinach, banana, and your number one natural products for a supplement-rich beginning.

Add seeds and nuts for surface and extra medical advantages.

Wellbeing Cognizant Choices for Weight Watchers

For those watching their weight, keeping a solid breakfast routine is fundamental. Here are a few choices customized to help you weigh the executive's objectives:

Egg White Veggie Omelet:

Low in calories yet high in protein.

Loaded with beautiful vegetables for added nutrients.

Chia Seed Pudding with New Natural Product:

Chia seeds give fiber and omega-3 unsaturated fats.

The new organic product adds regular pleasantness without an abundance of calories.

Quinoa Breakfast Bowl:

Quinoa is a finished protein, offering a delightful breakfast.

Top with new vegetables and a shower of olive oil for some zing.

Curds and Natural Product Bowl:

Curds are wealthy in protein and low in calories.

Match with your #1 natural products for a sweet and exquisite mix.

Family-Accommodating Breakfast Thoughts

Make mornings a glad family undertaking with these wonderful and healthy breakfast choices:

Banana Flapjacks:

Crush bananas into flapjack player for a normally sweet turn.

Top with berries and a spot of Greek yogurt.

Entire Grain French Toast Sticks:

Utilize entire grain bread for added fiber.

Ideal for little hands to plunge in maple syrup or yogurt.

Custom made Granola with Milk:

Make a custom granola blend with oats, nuts, and dried natural products.

Present with milk or yogurt for a crunchy and fulfilling dinner.

Peanut Butter Banana Toast:

Spread peanut butter on entire grain toast and top with banana cuts.

A straightforward, kid-accommodating choice with an equilibrium between protein and starches.

Whether you're a bustling proficient, a weight watcher, or a family searching for nutritious morning meals, these recipes take care of your particular requirements, guaranteeing your mornings start with a sound and stimulating lift.

Chapter 4: Mediterranean Lunch Bowls

Mediterranean Quinoa Power Bowl

Depiction: Stimulate your evening with a supplement-pressed quinoa bowl propelled by the Mediterranean. Loaded with protein and new veggies, it's an ideal equilibrium for a satisfying lunch.

Spending time in jail and Cooking Time: 30 minutes

Fixings:

1 cup quinoa, cooked

1 cup cherry tomatoes, divided

1 cucumber, diced

1/2 cup Kalamata olives, cut

1/4 cup red onion, finely cleaved

1/2 cup feta cheddar, disintegrated

New parsley, cleaved

Olive oil for sprinkling

Lemon wedges for decorating

Salt and pepper to taste

Directions:

In a bowl, join quinoa, cherry tomatoes, cucumber, olives, red onion, and feta cheddar.

Sprinkle olive oil over the combination and throw delicately to join.

Season with salt and pepper to taste.

Embellish with new parsley and present with lemon wedges as an afterthought.

2. Mediterranean Chickpea and Hummus Bowl

Portrayal: Submerge yourself in the goodness of chickpeas and the smoothness of hummus. This bowl is a protein-stuffed please motivated by Mediterranean flavors.

Spending time in jail and Cooking Time: 25 minutes

Fixings:

1 can chickpeas, depleted and flushed

1 tablespoon olive oil

1 teaspoon cumin

Salt and pepper to taste

1 cup cooked quinoa

1 cup cherry tomatoes, split

1 cucumber, cut

1/2 cup red chime pepper, diced

1/4 cup red onion, daintily cut

1/2 cup hummus

New parsley for decorating

Guidelines:

In a skillet, heat olive oil over medium intensity. Add chickpeas, cumin, salt, and pepper. Cook until chickpeas are brilliant brown.

In a bowl, orchestrate quinoa, cherry tomatoes, cucumber, red ringer pepper, and red onion.

Top the bowl with the cooked chickpeas.

Dab hummus as an afterthought and topping with new parsley.

3. Greek Plate of mixed greens with Barbecued Chicken Bowl

Portrayal: Transport yourself to the shores of Greece with this reviving bowl including an exemplary Greek serving of mixed greens and delicious barbecued chicken.

Spending time in jail and Cooking Time: 35 minutes

Fixings:

1 lb boneless, skinless chicken bosoms

1 tablespoon olive oil

1 teaspoon dried oregano

Salt and pepper to taste

4 cups blended greens

1 cup cherry tomatoes, divided

1 cucumber, diced

1/2 cup Kalamata olives, cut

1/2 cup feta cheddar, disintegrated

Greek dressing

Guidelines:

Rub chicken bosoms with olive oil, oregano, salt, and pepper. Barbecue until completely cooked.

Cut barbecued chicken into strips.

In a bowl, join blended greens, cherry tomatoes, cucumber, olives, and feta cheddar.

Top the serving of mixed greens with barbecued chicken tenders and sprinkle with Greek dressing.

4. Mediterranean Shrimp and Couscous Bowl

Portrayal: Plunge into a fish please with this Mediterranean bowl including delicious shrimp and cushy couscous.

Spending time in jail and Cooking Time: 20 minutes

Fixings:

1 lb shrimp, stripped and deveined

1 tablespoon olive oil

2 cloves garlic, minced

1 teaspoon paprika

Salt and pepper to taste

1 cup cooked couscous

1 cup cherry tomatoes, split

1/2 cup cucumber, diced

1/4 cup red onion, finely hacked

New mint for embellish

Directions:

In a skillet, heat olive oil over medium intensity. Add minced garlic, shrimp, paprika, salt, and pepper. Cook until shrimp are pink and obscure.

In a bowl, orchestrate couscous, cherry tomatoes, cucumber, and red onion.

Top the bowl with the cooked shrimp and trimming with new mint.

5. Mediterranean Lentil and Cooked Vegetable Bowl

Depiction: A generous and fulfilling bowl highlighting protein-rich lentils and a mixture of simmered vegetables for a healthy lunch insight.

Spending time in jail and Cooking Time: 40 minutes

Fixings:

1 cup dried lentils, cooked

2 cups blended vegetables (ringer peppers, zucchini, cherry tomatoes)

2 tablespoons olive oil

1 teaspoon dried thyme

Salt and pepper to taste

1 cup cooked bulgur

1/2 cup disintegrated goat cheddar

Balsamic coating for sprinkling

Guidelines:

Throw blended vegetables in with olive oil, dried thyme, salt, and pepper. Cook in the broiler until delicate.

In a bowl, layer cooked lentils, simmered vegetables, and cooked bulgur.

Sprinkle disintegrated goat cheddar over the bowl.

Sprinkle with balsamic coating before serving.

6. Mediterranean Fish and White Bean Bowl

Depiction: Experience the kinds of the Mediterranean with this protein-stuffed bowl highlighting fish, white beans, and a lively lemon dressing.

Spending time in jail and Cooking Time: 15 minutes

Fixings:

2 jars of fish, depleted

1 can white beans, depleted and washed

1/4 cup red onion, finely hacked

1/4 cup new parsley, hacked

2 tablespoons tricks

Zing and juice of one lemon

3 tablespoons olive oil

Salt and pepper to taste

Leafy greens for serving

Guidelines:

In a bowl, join fish, white beans, red onion, parsley, and tricks.

In a different little bowl, whisk together lemon zing, lemon juice, olive oil, salt, and pepper to make the dressing.

Pour the dressing over the fish blend and throw it delicately.

Serve over a bed of leafy greens.

7. Mediterranean Falafel and Tabouleh Bowl

Portrayal: Enjoy the credible kinds of the Mediterranean with a bowl highlighting firm falafel, new tabouleh, and a shower of tahini.

Spending time in jail and Cooking Time: 45 minutes

Fixings:

Locally acquired falafel (or hand-crafted)

1 cup tabouleh salad

1/2 cup cherry tomatoes, split

1/4 cup red onion, daintily cut

1/2 cucumber, diced

Tahini sauce for showering

New mint for embellish

Directions:

Prepare or sear falafel as per bundle directions.

In a bowl, organize tabouleh salad, cherry tomatoes, red onion, and cucumber.

Top the bowl with falafel.

8. Mediterranean Salmon and Orzo Bowl

Portrayal: Hoist your lunch with this choice bowl highlighting dish-burned salmon, lemony orzo, and a variety of energetic vegetables.

Spending time in jail and Cooking Time: 25 minutes

Fixings:

2 salmon filets

1 cup orzo, cooked

1 cup asparagus, cleaved

1/2 cup cherry tomatoes, split

1/4 cup feta cheddar, disintegrated

Zing and juice of one lemon

2 tablespoons olive oil

New dill for decorating

Salt and pepper to taste

Directions:

Season salmon filets with salt, pepper, and a press of lemon juice. Skillet singe until completely cooked.

In a bowl, join cooked orzo, asparagus, cherry tomatoes, and feta cheddar.

Put the burned salmon on top of the orzo blend.

Shower with olive oil, sprinkle lemon zing and topping with new dill.

9. Mediterranean Eggplant and Hummus Bowl

Depiction: Drench yourself in the rich kinds of cooked eggplant matched with velvety hummus in this wonderful veggie lover well-disposed lunch bowl.

Spending time in jail and Cooking Time: 30 minutes

Fixings:

1 enormous eggplant, cut

2 tablespoons olive oil

1 teaspoon smoked paprika

Salt and pepper to taste

1 cup cooked quinoa

1/2 cup hummus

1/4 cup cherry tomatoes, split

1/4 cup red onion, daintily cut

New parsley for embellish

Directions:

Preheat the stove to 400°F (200°C).

Throw eggplant cuts with olive oil, smoked paprika, salt, and pepper. Broil until brilliant and delicate.

In a bowl, layer cooked quinoa, broiled eggplant, cherry tomatoes, and red onion.

Dab hummus as an afterthought and trimming with new parsley.

10. Mediterranean Turkey and Spinach Bowl

Depiction: Partake in a lean and protein-pressed lunch bowl highlighting prepared ground turkey, sautéed spinach, and an eruption of Mediterranean flavors.

Spending time in jail and Cooking Time: 20 minutes

Fixings:

1 lb ground turkey

1 tablespoon olive oil

1 teaspoon dried oregano

2 cups of new spinach

1 cup cooked couscous

1/2 cup cherry tomatoes, split

1/4 cup feta cheddar, disintegrated

Lemon wedges for embellish

Salt and pepper to taste

Guidelines:

In a skillet, heat olive oil over medium intensity. Add ground turkey, dried oregano, salt, and pepper. Cook until turkey is caramelized.

In a similar skillet, add new spinach and sauté until withered.

In a bowl, layer cooked couscous, prepared turkey, sautéed spinach, cherry tomatoes, and feta cheddar.

Present with lemon wedges as an afterthought for a lively touch.

Helpful and Heavenly Lunch Choices for Wellness Lovers

In the high-speed world we live in, finding the ideal harmony between comfort and sustenance is vital, particularly for those committed to keeping a sound and fit way of life. Feast preparing has arisen as a distinct advantage, permitting people to assume command over their sustenance without settling on taste. We should investigate a scope of helpful and delectable lunch choices intended for feast preppers, with an extraordinary accentuation on giving adjusted and nutritious decisions to wellness lovers.

1. Barbecued Chicken Quinoa Bowl

Fixings: Barbecued chicken bosom, tri-variety quinoa, blended vegetables, avocado cuts, and a shower of olive oil.

Benefits: Loaded with lean protein, fundamental fats, and fiber from quinoa, this bowl powers your body for ideal execution.

2. Salmon and Yam Hash

Fixings: Heated salmon lumps, broiled yams, sautéed spinach, cherry tomatoes, and a sprinkle of chia seeds.

Benefits: Plentiful in omega-3 unsaturated fats, nutrients, and minerals, this dish upholds muscle recuperation and by and large prosperity.

3. Mediterranean Chickpea Salad

Fixings: Chickpeas, cherry tomatoes, cucumber, red onion, feta cheddar, olives, and a lemon vinaigrette.

Benefits: High in plant-based protein and cell reinforcements, this reviving serving of mixed greens gives supported energy to your exercises.

4. Turkey and Quinoa Stuffed Peppers

Fixings: Ground turkey, quinoa, dark beans, corn, diced tomatoes, and taco preparing, heated in chime peppers.

Benefits: A protein-stuffed, low-carb choice that guides in muscle working while at the same time holding your carb consumption under tight restraints.

5. Shrimp and Avocado Wrap

Fixings: Barbecued shrimp, entire grain wrap, blended greens, cherry tomatoes, and a velvety avocado dressing.

Benefits: A light yet fulfilling choice, wealthy in lean protein, solid fats, and fiber, ideal for post-exercise recuperation.

Tips for Ideal Dinner Preparing:

Segment Control: Guarantee an equilibrium of macronutrients by controlling piece sizes as indicated by your wellness objectives.

Various Fixings: Integrate different brilliant vegetables, lean proteins, entire grains, and solid fats for a balanced feast.

Prep in Bunches: Smooth out your feast prep by cooking in bigger amounts and distributing them into individual holders for the week.

Dinner preparation isn't just about saving time; it's tied in with settling on purposeful decisions to fuel your body for progress. These helpful and flavorful lunch choices take special care of the bustling person as well as focus on the dietary necessities of wellness lovers, adding to a balanced and reasonable way to deal with solid living. Hoist your lunch game and make a stride nearer to accomplishing your wellness objectives with these delightful and nutritious recipes.

Chapter 5: Family Dinners Made Easy

Title: Mediterranean Chicken Paella

Portrayal/History: A one-skillet wonder motivated by the exuberant soul of Mediterranean family social events. This paella unites delicate chicken, tasty saffron rice, and a variety of bright vegetables.

Spending time in jail and Cooking Time: Serves 4; Planning Time: 15 minutes, Cook Time: 30 minutes

Fixings:

1 lb boneless, skinless chicken thighs, diced

2 cups paella rice

1 onion, finely hacked

2 chime peppers (ideally red and yellow), cut

1 cup cherry tomatoes, split

3 cloves garlic, minced

4 cups chicken stock

1 teaspoon saffron strings

1 teaspoon paprika

Salt and pepper to taste

Olive oil

Directions:

In a huge paella container, sauté chicken in olive oil until cooked. Eliminate and save.

In a similar skillet, sauté onions and garlic until relaxed.

Add rice, saffron, paprika, and mix to cover in the oil.

Pour in chicken stock and bring to a stew.

Orchestrate chicken, chime peppers, and tomatoes uniformly on top of the rice.

Cover and stew for 20-25 minutes until the rice is cooked and the chicken is delicate.

Season with salt and pepper to taste. Serve hot.

Title: Lemon Spice Prepared Salmon

Portrayal/Origin story: A reviving and nutritious dish that easily carries the flavor of the Mediterranean to your family supper table. The blend of lively lemon and sweet-smelling spices upgrades the normal kinds of salmon.

Spending time in jail and Cooking Time: Serves 4; Planning Time: 10 minutes, Cook Time: 20 minutes

Fixings:

4 salmon filets

2 lemons, cut

3 tablespoons olive oil

2 cloves garlic, minced

1 tablespoon new dill, hacked

1 tablespoon new parsley, hacked

Salt and pepper to taste

Directions:

Preheat stove to 375°F (190°C).

Put salmon filets on a baking sheet fixed with material paper.

Shower olive oil over the salmon, guaranteeing an even coat.

Sprinkle minced garlic, dill, and parsley over the filets.

Orchestrate lemon cuts on top of each filet.

Season with salt and pepper.

Prepare for 15-20 minutes or until salmon drops effectively with a fork. Serve hot.

Title: Vegetable Pesto Pasta Joy

Portrayal/History: A vivid and healthy pasta dish that commends the overflow of Mediterranean vegetables. The fragrant pesto sauce integrates the flavors, making a wonderful family-accommodating feast.

Spending time in jail and Cooking Time: Serves 4; Planning Time: 20 minutes, Cook Time: 15 minutes

Fixings:

8 oz penne pasta

1 cup cherry tomatoes, split

1 zucchini, daintily cut

1 cup broccoli florets

1/2 cup dark olives, cut

1/4 cup pine nuts, toasted

1/2 cup ground Parmesan cheddar

1 cup new basil leaves

2 cloves garlic

1/2 cup additional virgin olive oil

Salt and pepper to taste

Guidelines:

Cook pasta as indicated by bundle guidelines. Channel and put away.

In a food processor, mix basil, garlic, pine nuts, and Parmesan cheddar.

While mixing, gradually add olive oil until a smooth pesto sauce structures.

In a huge dish, sauté zucchini, cherry tomatoes, and broccoli until delicate.

Add cooked pasta to the container and throw with the vegetable blend.

Pour the pesto sauce over the pasta and vegetables, guaranteeing in any event, covering.

Mix in cut olives and season with salt and pepper. Serve warm.

Title: Barbecued Mediterranean Chicken Sticks

Portrayal/Origin story: Imbued with Mediterranean flavors, these barbecued chicken sticks are a hit for family suppers. The blend of marinated chicken and energetic veggies conveys a delightful and good dinner.

Spending time in jail and Cooking Time: Serves 4; Planning Time: 25 minutes (in addition to marinating time), Cook Time: 15 minutes

Fixings:

1.5 lbs boneless, skinless chicken bosoms, cut into blocks

1 red onion, cut into lumps

1 red ringer pepper, cut into pieces

1 yellow ringer pepper, cut into pieces

1/4 cup olive oil

2 tablespoons lemon juice

3 cloves garlic, minced

1 teaspoon dried oregano

1 teaspoon ground cumin

Salt and pepper to taste

Directions:

In a bowl, whisk together olive oil, lemon juice, minced garlic, oregano, cumin, salt, and pepper.

Add chicken blocks to the marinade, they are very much covered to guarantee they. Marinate for no less than 60 minutes.

Preheat the barbecue to medium-high intensity.

String marinated chicken, onion, and chime peppers onto sticks.

Barbecue sticks for 12-15 minutes, turning incidentally, until chicken is cooked through and veggies are scorched.

Serve the sticks hot with your number one side dishes.

Title: Quinoa Stuffed Chime Peppers

Portrayal/History: Lift your family supper with these Mediterranean-motivated quinoa-stuffed ringer peppers. Loaded with protein and vivid vegetables, this dish is both nutritious and outwardly engaging.

Spending time in jail and Cooking Time: Serves 4; Planning Time: 30 minutes, Cook Time: 25 minutes

Fixings:

4 huge chime peppers, split, and seeds eliminated

1 cup quinoa, cooked

1 can (15 oz) chickpeas, depleted and flushed

1 cup cherry tomatoes, diced

1/2 cup feta cheddar, disintegrated

1/4 cup Kalamata olives, slashed

1/4 cup new parsley, slashed

1 teaspoon dried oregano

Salt and pepper to taste

Olive oil for showering

Directions:

Preheat the stove to 375°F (190°C).

In a huge bowl, blend cooked quinoa, chickpeas, cherry tomatoes, feta, olives, parsley, oregano, salt, and pepper.

Stuff each chime pepper half with the quinoa blend.

Shower olive oil over the stuffed peppers and place them in a baking dish.

Heat for 25 minutes or until the peppers are delicate.

Decorate with extra parsley and feta before serving.

Title: Eggplant Parmesan Rolls

Depiction/Origin Story: A Mediterranean bend on an exemplary dish, these eggplant parmesan rolls consolidate the extravagance of eggplant with exquisite marinara sauce and softened cheddar, making an encouraging family supper.

Spending time in jail and Cooking Time: Serves 4; Planning Time: 20 minutes, Cook Time: 30 minutes

Fixings:

2 huge eggplants, meagerly cut longwise

1 cup ricotta cheddar

1/2 cup ground Parmesan cheddar

1 egg, beaten

2 cups marinara sauce

1 cup mozzarella cheddar, destroyed

New basil leaves for embellish

Salt and pepper to taste

Olive oil for brushing

Guidelines:

Preheat the broiler to 375°F (190°C).

Brush eggplant cuts with olive oil and season with salt and pepper.

Barbecue or cook the eggplant cuts until delicate, around 3 minutes for every side.

In a bowl, consolidate ricotta, Parmesan, and beaten egg.

Spread a spoonful of the cheddar blend onto every eggplant cut, then roll them up.

In a baking dish, spread a fair layer of marinara sauce.

Place the eggplant rolls crease side down in the dish, top with outstanding marinara sauce, and sprinkle with mozzarella.

Heat for 25-30 minutes or until the cheddar is softened and effervescent. Embellish with new basil before serving.

Title: Greek Lemon Garlic Broil Chicken

Portrayal/Origin story: Transport your family to the Greek wide open with this delicious dish of chicken implanted with fiery lemon and fragrant garlic. A basic yet noteworthy dish ideal for Sunday suppers.

Spending time in jail and Cooking Time: Serves 4; Planning Time: 15 minutes, Cook Time: 60 minutes

Fixings:

1 entire chicken (around 4 lbs)

4 lemons, squeezed and zing of 2 lemons

6 cloves garlic, minced

2 tablespoons new oregano, slashed

1/4 cup olive oil

Salt and pepper to taste

1 cup chicken stock

Guidelines:

Preheat the broiler to 375°F (190°C).

In a bowl, blend lemon juice, lemon zing, minced garlic, oregano, olive oil, salt, and pepper.

Wipe the chicken off and rub the lemon-garlic blend everywhere and inside the cavity.

Place the chicken in a broiling dish and empty the chicken stock into the skillet.

Broil for roughly 1 hour or until the inward temperature comes to 165°F (74°C).

Season the chicken with dish squeezes like clockwork.

Let the chicken rest for 10 minutes before cutting. Present with cooked vegetables or potatoes.

Title: Mediterranean Shrimp and Couscous Skillet

Depiction/Origin story: A fast and tasty dish that consolidates succulent shrimp, cushy couscous, and a mixture of

Mediterranean flavors. Ideal for occupied weeknights when you need a quarrel-free yet fulfilling feast.

Spending time in jail and Cooking Time: Serves 4; Planning Time: 15 minutes, Cook Time: 20 minutes

Fixings:

1 lb huge shrimp, stripped and deveined

1 cup couscous, cooked

1 red chime pepper, diced

1 yellow chime pepper, diced

1 cup cherry tomatoes, split

3 cloves garlic, minced

1 teaspoon cumin

1 teaspoon smoked paprika

1/2 teaspoon red pepper chips (discretionary)

New parsley for embellish

Olive oil for cooking

Directions:

In a huge skillet, heat olive oil over medium intensity.

Add shrimp and cook until pink, around 2-3 minutes for each side. Eliminate shrimp and put it away.

In a similar skillet, sauté garlic, chime peppers, and cherry tomatoes until relaxed.

Mix in cumin, smoked paprika, and red pepper chips.

Add cooked couscous and shrimp back to the skillet. Throw until all around joined and warmed through.

Embellish with new parsley before serving.

Title: Mediterranean Stuffed Zucchini Boats

Depiction/History: These zucchini boats are a magnificent and nutritious method for getting a charge out of Mediterranean flavors. Loaded with a combination of ground turkey, quinoa, and lively veggies, this dish is both fulfilling and solid.

Spending time in jail and Cooking Time: Serves 4; Planning Time: 25 minutes, Cook Time: 25 minutes

Fixings:

4 enormous zucchini, split the long way

1/2 lb ground turkey

1 cup cooked quinoa

1 onion, finely slashed

1 ringer pepper, diced

1 cup cherry tomatoes, diced

2 cloves garlic, minced

1 teaspoon dried oregano

1 teaspoon ground cumin

Salt and pepper to taste

Feta cheddar for embellish

Olive oil for cooking

Guidelines:

Preheat the broiler to 375°F (190°C).

Scoop out the focal point of every zucchini half to make a boat-like shape.

In a skillet, heat olive oil and sauté onion and garlic until mellowed.

Add ground turkey and cook until seared.

Mix in diced chime pepper, cherry tomatoes, oregano, cumin, salt, and pepper. Cook for 5 extra minutes.

Blend in cooked quinoa and stuff the zucchini boats with the turkey combination.

Heat for 20-25 minutes or until the zucchini is delicate.

Decorate with disintegrated feta before serving.

Title: Caprese Stuffed Chicken Bosoms

Depiction/History: Lift your family supper with these heavenly Caprese-stuffed chicken bosoms. Overflowing with the kinds of new tomatoes, mozzarella, and basil, this dish is a genuine festival of Mediterranean effortlessness.

Spending time in jail and Cooking Time: Serves 4; Planning Time: 15 minutes, Cook Time: 30 minutes

Fixings:

4 boneless, skinless chicken bosoms

1 cup cherry tomatoes, cut

1 cup new mozzarella, cut

1/2 cup new basil leaves

2 tablespoons balsamic coating

Salt and pepper to taste

Olive oil for showering

Directions:

Preheat the stove to 375°F (190°C).

Cut a pocket into every chicken bosom without carving the whole way through.

Season the chicken with salt and pepper.

Stuff each pocket with cherry tomatoes, mozzarella, and new basil.

Shower olive oil over the stuffed chicken bosoms.

Prepare for 25-30 minutes or until the chicken is cooked through.

Shower balsamic coating over the top before serving.

Raising Family Suppers with Mediterranean Style

In the rushing about of our day-to-day routines, family meals act as a holy future time together, share stories, and feed both body and soul. Raise your family's feasting experience with these tasty supper recipes imbued with the energetic and healthy kinds of the Mediterranean. Whether you're a carefully prepared cook or a kitchen beginner, these dishes are intended to give pleasure and a dash of refinement to your family table.

1. Mediterranean Chicken with Lemon and Olives:

Delicious chicken thighs marinated in a mix of olive oil, lemon, garlic, and a variety of Mediterranean spices.

Family-accommodating tip: Present with couscous or quinoa for a generous and nutritious bend.

2. Heated Mediterranean Fish Parcels:

New fish filets joined with cherry tomatoes, Kalamata olives, and artichoke hearts, enveloped by material paper and heated flawlessly.

Dietary adaptability: Effectively versatile for sans gluten or without dairy inclinations.

3. Veggie-stacked Greek Serving of mixed greens Pita Wraps:

Fresh veggies, feta cheddar, and a fiery natively constructed tzatziki sauce got into entire wheat pitas.

Dietary choices: Ideal for vegans and effectively adaptable sans gluten consuming fewer calories with the best selection of wraps.

4. Quinoa Stuffed Chime Peppers with Feta:

Beautiful chime peppers loaded up with a nutritious blend of quinoa, chickpeas, and feta cheddar.

Dietary inclusivity: Ideal for veggie lovers and without gluten counts calories, offering a healthy and fulfilling choice.

5. Mediterranean Lentil Soup:

An encouraging and nutritious mix of lentils, tomatoes, spinach, and a touch of cumin.

Dietary contemplations: Normally vegetarian and sans gluten, settling on a comprehensive decision for different dietary limitations.

6. Barbecued Veggie and Halloumi Sticks:

Burned flawlessness of zucchini, cherry tomatoes, and halloumi cheddar sprinkled with a balsamic coating.

Dietary flexibility: Reasonable for veggie lovers and effectively movable for sans lactose inclinations.

7. Spinach and Feta Stuffed Chicken Bosom:

Succulent chicken bosoms loaded up with a magnificent combination of spinach and feta, making an eruption of Mediterranean flavors.

Choices for dietary limitations: Low-carb and without gluten, taking special care of different dietary necessities.

Implant your family suppers with the glow of Mediterranean accommodation and relish the healthy decency of these painstakingly created recipes. Whether you're taking care of dietary limitations or just intending to entice taste buds, these dishes vow to make each family feast a remarkable culinary excursion. Assemble around the table, share chuckling, and let the Mediterranean appeal change your feasting experience.

Chapter 6: Joyful Snacking with Mediterranean Flair

1 Title: Olive Tapenade Crostini

Depiction: A magnificent hors d'oeuvre propelled by Mediterranean flavors, highlighting a strong olive tapenade on fresh crostini.

Serving Size: 12 pieces

Planning Time: 15 minutes

Cooking Time: 10 minutes

Fixings:

1 cup dark olives, pitted

1/4 cup tricks

2 cloves garlic

2 tablespoons new lemon juice

1/4 cup additional virgin olive oil

Loaf cut

Directions:

In a food processor, consolidate olives, escapades, garlic, and lemon juice. Beat until finely hacked.

With the processor running, shower in olive oil until a smooth glue structure.

Toast roll cuts and spread olive tapenade on top.

2. Title: Greek Yogurt Cucumber Cups

Portrayal: A reviving nibble with a Mediterranean wind, these cucumber cups are loaded up with a lively Greek yogurt combination.

Serving Size: 6 cups

Planning Time: 20 minutes

Cooking Time: 0 minutes

Fixings:

2 cucumbers, stripped and cut

1 cup Greek yogurt

1 tablespoon new dill, slashed

1 tablespoon lemon juice

Salt and pepper to taste

Directions:

Scoop out the focal point of cucumber cuts to make cups.

In a bowl, blend Greek yogurt, dill, lemon squeeze, salt, and pepper.

Fill cucumber cups with the yogurt blend.

3. Title: Stuffed Grape Leaves (Dolma)

Portrayal: An exemplary Mediterranean dish, these stuffed grape leaves are loaded up with a delightful rice and spice blend.

Serving Size: 24 pieces

Planning Time: 30 minutes

Cooking Time: 45 minutes

Fixings:

1 cup grape leaves, safeguarded in salt water

1 cup long-grain rice

1/4 cup pine nuts

1/4 cup new mint, slashed

1/4 cup new parsley, slashed

1/4 cup lemon juice

2 tablespoons olive oil

Directions:

Wash grape leaves and whiten them in steaming hot water.

In a bowl, blend rice, pine nuts, mint, parsley, lemon juice, and olive oil.

Put a spoonful of the blend on every grape leaf and roll firmly.

4. Title: Hummus and Cooked Red Pepper Pita Pockets

Portrayal: A fast and simple bite highlighting the exemplary blend of hummus and cooked red peppers in a pocket-sized enchant.

Serving Size: 4 pockets

Planning Time: 10 minutes

Cooking Time: 0 minutes

Fixings:

1 cup hummus

1/2 cup simmered red peppers, cut

4 entire wheat pita pockets

Guidelines:

Warm pita pockets in a toaster oven or broiler.

Spread hummus inside each pocket.

Stuff with cuts of simmered red peppers.

5. Title: Mediterranean Veggie Sticks

Depiction: Bright and delightful veggie sticks including various Mediterranean vegetables and a fiery marinade.

Serving Size: 8 sticks

Planning Time: 20 minutes

Cooking Time: 15 minutes

Fixings:

2 zucchinis, cut

1 16 ounces cherry tomatoes

1 red onion, cut into lumps

1 ringer pepper, cut into lumps

1/4 cup olive oil

2 cloves garlic, minced

1 teaspoon dried oregano

Salt and pepper to taste

Directions:

Preheat the barbecue or stove.

String vegetables onto sticks.

Blend olive oil, garlic, oregano, salt, and pepper. Brush over sticks and barbecue until veggies are delicate.

6. Title: Feta and Spinach Stuffed Mushrooms

Depiction: These flavorful stuffed mushrooms are loaded up with a combination of feta cheddar and spinach, making a scaled-down charm.

Serving Size: 16 mushrooms

Planning Time: 25 minutes

Cooking Time: 20 minutes

Fixings:

16 huge mushrooms, stems eliminated

1 cup feta cheddar, disintegrated

1 cup new spinach, hacked

2 cloves garlic, minced

2 tablespoons olive oil

Directions:

Preheat the stove to 375°F (190°C).

In a bowl, consolidate feta, spinach, and garlic.

Stuff each mushroom cap with the blend, shower with olive oil, and heat until brilliant.

7. Title: Tzatziki and Pita Chip Platter

Portrayal: A group-satisfying platter including hand-crafted tzatziki and fresh heated pita chips for plunging.

Serving Size: 6 servings

Planning Time: 15 minutes

Cooking Time: 10 minutes

Fixings:

1 cup Greek yogurt

1 cucumber, finely diced

2 cloves garlic, minced

1 tablespoon new dill, hacked

Salt and pepper to taste

6 pita bread adjusts, cut into triangles

Directions:

Blend Greek yogurt, cucumber, garlic, dill, salt, and pepper to make tzatziki.

Heat pita triangles until fresh.

Serve the tzatziki close by the pita chips.

8. Title: Mediterranean Cheddar Board

Depiction: A modern yet basic cheddar board highlighting a choice of Mediterranean cheeses, olives, and dried natural products.

Serving Size: 4 servings

Planning Time: 15 minutes

Cooking Time: 0 minutes

Fixings:

200g feta cheddar

150g manchego cheddar

1 cup blended olives

1/2 cup dried apricots

1/4 cup honey

Guidelines:

Organize cheeses, olives, and dried natural products on a platter.

Shower honey over the feta.

Present with dried-up bread or wafers.

9. Title: Lemon Garlic Edamame

Portrayal: A sound and tasty bend on edamame, implanted with the splendor of lemon and the glow of garlic.

Serving Size: 4 servings

Planning Time: 10 minutes

Cooking Time: 5 minutes

Fixings:

2 cups edamame, defrosted whenever frozen

2 tablespoons olive oil

Zing of 1 lemon

2 cloves garlic, minced

Salt to taste

Directions:

Bubble edamame for 3-5 minutes, then channel.

In a dish, sauté garlic in olive oil until fragrant.

Add edamame, lemon zing, and salt. Throw until all around covered.

10. Title: Pistachio and Honey Granola Bars

Portrayal: A healthy and energy-supporting tidbit including the nutty decency of pistachios and the regular pleasantness of honey.

Serving Size: 12 bars

Planning Time: 15 minutes

Cooking Time: 20 minutes

Fixings:

2 cups moved oats

1 cup pistachios, hacked

1/2 cup honey

1/4 cup coconut oil

1/2 cup dried cranberries

1 teaspoon vanilla concentrate

Touch of salt

Directions:

Preheat the stove to 350°F (175°C) and line a baking dish with material paper.

In a huge bowl, join moved oats, slashed pistachios, dried cranberries, and salt.

In a little pot, dissolve honey and coconut oil. Eliminate from intensity and mix in vanilla concentrate.

Pour the wet blend over the dry fixings and blend well.

Press the blend into the pre-arranged baking dish and heat for 20 minutes or until brilliant.

Permit to cool prior to cutting into bars.

Lift Your Health: Supplement Rich Nibble Thoughts for Each Way of Life

In our speedy world, finding the right harmony between well-being and comfort is fundamental. For health searchers, occupied experts, and those going for the gold, picking snacks carefully can have a massive effect on in general prosperity. Here is a manual for tasty and nutritious nibble thoughts custom-made to your particular necessities.

Solid Nibble Thoughts for Health Searchers:

Nut and Seed Blend:

Consolidate almonds, pecans, pumpkin seeds, and a dash of dull chocolate for a fantastic blend of solid fats and cell reinforcements.

Greek Yogurt Parfait:

Layer Greek yogurt with new berries, granola, and a shower of honey for a protein-stuffed, delightful treat.

Veggie Sticks with Hummus:

Partake in the mash of beautiful ringer peppers, carrots, and cucumber with a side of hummus, giving a portion of fiber and nutrients.

Quinoa Salad Cups:

Plan quinoa salad cups with cherry tomatoes, feta cheddar, and a sprinkle of spices for a reviving and healthy bite.

Chia Pudding:

Blend chia seeds with almond milk and allow it to sit for the time being. Top with cut leafy foods and a sprinkle of nuts for a magnificent pudding.

Segment Controlled Snacks for Weight The executives:

Air-Popped Popcorn:

Fulfill your desire for mash with air-popped popcorn, prepared with a touch of healthful yeast or your #1 flavors.

Dim Chocolate Covered Almonds:

Partake in a sweet and exquisite mix by covering almonds with dim chocolate, giving cell reinforcements and sound fats.

Hard-Bubbled Eggs:

A magnificent wellspring of protein, hard-bubbled eggs are not difficult to plan and advantageous for segment control.

Edamame Units:

Steam edamame cases and daintily salt them for a protein-pressed, fiber-rich bite that assists with satiety.

Prepared Yam Chips:

Cut yams daintily, throw with olive oil and prepare until fresh for a delicious option in contrast to conventional chips.

Light meals for Occupied Experts in a hurry:

Protein Smoothies:

Mix your #1 organic products, a scoop of protein powder, and a modest bunch of spinach for a nutritious and convenient smoothie.

Trail Blend Packs:

Plan individual packs of trail blend in with a blend of nuts, dried organic products, and seeds for a speedy jolt of energy.

Nut Margarine and Banana Sandwich:

Spread almond or peanut butter on entire-grain bread and add banana cuts for a fantastic and filling nibble.

String Cheddar and Grapes:

Match string cheddar with a modest bunch of grapes for a helpful and adjusted blend of protein and normal sugars.

Vegetable Sushi Rolls:

Make speedy vegetable sushi rolls utilizing nori sheets, avocado, cucumber, and your number one veggies for a versatile and nutritious chomp.

By integrating these nibble thoughts into your everyday schedule, you can hoist your well-being process, deal with your weight successfully, and stay aware of the requests of a bustling way of life. Keep in mind, that little, careful decisions can prompt critical enhancements in your general well-being and imperativeness.

Chapter 7: Indulgent yet Nourishing Desserts

Chocolate Avocado Mousse

Depiction: A rich and smooth chocolate mousse that conceals confidentiality - the smoothness comes from ready avocados!
Serving Size: 4
Planning Time: 15 minutes
Cooking Time: 0 minutes

Fixings:

2 ready avocados
1/2 cup cocoa powder
1/4 cup maple syrup
1 tsp vanilla concentrate
Touch of salt
1/4 cup almond milk

Directions:

Scoop out avocado tissue into a blender.

Add cocoa powder, maple syrup, vanilla concentrate, salt, and almond milk.

Mix until smooth and velvety.

Refrigerate for somewhere around 2 hours prior to serving.

2. Banana Nutella Crepes

Depiction: A wonderful blend of slim crepes loaded up with cut bananas and a liberal spread of Nutella.

Serving Size: 6 crepes

Planning Time: 20 minutes

Cooking Time: 15 minutes

Fixings:

1 cup regular baking flour

2 eggs

1 cup milk

Spot of salt

3 ready bananas, cut

Nutella

Slashed hazelnuts to decorate

Guidelines:

In a bowl, whisk flour, eggs, milk, and salt until smooth.

Heat a non-stick skillet and pour a spoon of player, whirling to equitably cover the container.

Cook until edges are brilliant, flip, and cook the opposite side.

Spread Nutella on each crepe, add banana cuts, crease, and sprinkle with cleaved hazelnuts.

3. Chia Seed Pudding Parfait

Portrayal: A faultless pleasure with layers of chia seed pudding, new berries, and granola.

Serving Size: 2 parfaits

Planning Time: 10 minutes + short-term chilling

Cooking Time: 0 minutes

Fixings:

1/4 cup chia seeds

1 cup almond milk

1 tbsp maple syrup

1 cup blended berries

1/2 cup granola

Guidelines:

Blend chia seeds, almond milk, and maple syrup in a container, and refrigerate for the time being.

In serving glasses, layer chia pudding, new berries, and granola.

Rehash layers and top with additional berries.

4. Pumpkin Flavor Energy Nibbles

Depiction: Reduced down joy joining the kinds of pumpkin and warming flavors for a nutritious treat.

Serving Size: 12 nibbles

Planning Time: 15 minutes

Cooking Time: 0 minutes

Fixings:

1 cup moved oats

1/2 cup pumpkin puree

1/4 cup almond margarine

1/4 cup honey

1 tsp pumpkin zest

1/2 cup destroyed coconut (for rolling)

Guidelines:

Blend oats, pumpkin puree, almond margarine, honey, and pumpkin zest in a bowl.

Roll into reduced down balls.

Roll each ball in destroyed coconut.

Chill in the cooler for 30 minutes before serving.

5. Coconut Chocolate-Plunged Strawberries

Portrayal: Succulent strawberries dunked in dull chocolate and moved in destroyed coconut for a tropical contort.

Serving Size: 12 strawberries

Planning Time: 20 minutes

Cooking Time: 5 minutes

Fixings:

12 new strawberries, washed and dried

1 cup dull chocolate chips

1/2 cup destroyed coconut

Directions:

Dissolve chocolate chips in a microwave-safe bowl.

Dunk every strawberry into softened chocolate, covering half of the berry.

Roll the chocolate-shrouded part in the destroyed coconut.

Put on a material-lined plate and refrigerate until chocolate sets.

6. Almond Margarine Stuffed Dates

Depiction: A straightforward yet wanton treat including dates loaded down with rich almond margarine.

Serving Size: 10 dates

Planning Time: 10 minutes

Cooking Time: 0 minutes

Fixings:

10 Medjool dates, pitted

1/4 cup almond margarine

Ocean salt (discretionary)

Guidelines:

Painstakingly cut each date and eliminate the pit.

Fill each date with a teaspoon of almond margarine.

Alternatively, sprinkle a spot of ocean salt on top.

Chill in the fridge for 30 minutes before serving.

7. Raspberry Chocolate Greek Yogurt Parfait

Depiction: Layers of rich Greek yogurt, tart raspberry compote, and dim chocolate make this parfait a great and nutritious pastry.

Serving Size: 2 parfaits

Planning Time: 15 minutes

Cooking Time: 10 minutes

Fixings:

2 cups Greek yogurt

1 cup new or frozen raspberries

2 tbsp honey

1/4 cup dim chocolate, cleaved

Guidelines:

In a pan, cook raspberries and honey until they structure a compote.

In serving glasses, layer Greek yogurt, raspberry compote, and hacked dull chocolate.

Rehash layers and get done with a sprinkle of chocolate on top.

8. Oats Raisin Treat Batter Chomps
Portrayal: The nostalgic kinds of oats raisin treats in a sound, no-prepare, scaled-down structure.
Serving Size: 15 chomps
Planning Time: 15 minutes
Cooking Time: 0 minutes
Fixings:
1 cup moved oats
1/2 cup raisins
1/4 cup almond margarine
2 tbsp honey
1 tsp vanilla concentrate
1/2 tsp cinnamon
Guidelines:
Mix moved oats and raisins in a food processor until finely slashed.
Add almond margarine, honey, vanilla concentrate, and cinnamon. Beat until very much joined.
Fold the combination into reduced down balls.
Chill in the cooler for no less than 30 minutes before serving

9. **Mango Coconut Rice Pudding**

Portrayal: Rich coconut rice pudding finished off with new mango for a tropical curve on an exemplary sweet.

Serving Size: 4

Planning Time: 10 minutes

Cooking Time: 25 minutes

Fixings:

1 cup Arborio rice

2 cups coconut milk

1/4 cup sugar

1 tsp vanilla concentrate

1 ready mango, diced

Directions:

In a pot, consolidate rice, coconut milk, and sugar. Cook until the rice is delicate.

Mix in vanilla concentrate.

Partition the pudding into serving bowls and top with diced mango.

10. Matcha Green Tea Pleasant Cream

Portrayal: A reviving and sound choice to frozen yogurt, this pleasant cream is mixed with gritty kinds of matcha.

Serving Size: 4

Planning Time: 10 minutes + freezing

Cooking Time: 0 minutes

Fixings:

4 ready bananas, cut and frozen

1 tsp matcha powder

1/4 cup coconut milk

Pistachios for embellish

Directions:

Mix frozen banana cuts, matcha powder, and coconut milk until smooth.

Move to a cooler safe compartment and freeze for something like 2 hours.

Scoop into bowls and embellishment with cleaved pistachios.

Sweet treats with an emphasis on well-being cognizant fixings

Enjoying sweet treats doesn't need to be an indulgence; it tends to be a magnificent encounter that lines up with well-being cognizant decisions.

Find the ideal harmony between balance, fulfillment, and careful fixings with our determination of heavenly treats custom-made for Weight Watchers and appropriate for family social events.

Embracing Wellbeing Cognizant Fixings

Our sweet treats are created with extreme attention to detail, highlighting healthy and supplement rich fixings. From almond flour to coconut sugar, we focus on choices that add a healthful lift to your extravagance. These treats avoid counterfeit added substances, zeroing in on normal pleasantness and goodness without settling on taste.

Control: The Way to Virtuous Happiness

For weight watchers, control is the foundation of a feasible and charming excursion. Our sweet treats are divided flawlessly, permitting you to savor each chomp without the concern of crashing your well-being objectives. Relish the flavors while keeping focused on your health goals - it's a sweet triumph for your taste buds and your waistline.

Dessert Choices for Families and Social events

Make enduring recollections with our treatment choices appropriate for family get-togethers. From cozy suppers to merry festivals, our reach takes care of assorted preferences and inclinations. Look over a variety of righteous enjoyments that enticement for both the well-being cognizant and those with a sweet tooth, guaranteeing everybody around the table tracks down a treat to relish.

An Orchestra of Flavors and Surfaces

Our assortment brags an orchestra of flavors and surfaces, from rich dull chocolate guilty pleasures to fruity joys. Every pastry is fastidiously created to give a wonderful encounter that goes past pleasantness. Investigate the creativity of taste with treats that are outwardly engaging as well as tempting to the sense of taste.

Supporting Body and Soul

Lift your treat insight by embracing choices that support both body and soul. Fixings like cell-reinforcement pressed berries and heart-solid nuts add to the general prosperity, making your sweet minutes something beyond a temporary delight. It's a cognizant decision to treat yourself with pastries that line up with your well-being process.

All in all, our sweet treats rethink the pastry experience, consolidating the domains of extravagance and health. Whether you're a weight watcher searching for control, a parent taking care of family tastes, or a host planning for a get-together, our sweets guarantee a superb excursion for your taste buds while remembering well-being. Embrace the pleasantness of existence with treats that are as great for your body as they are for your spirit.

Chapter 8: Celebrating Mediterranean Holidays

Embrace the lavishness of Mediterranean culture and culinary enjoyment with Section 8, an excursion into the core of festivity through unique event recipes, dinner thoughts, and an all-encompassing way to deal with prosperity. This section is a dining experience for foodies and social pioneers the same, offering an embroidery of flavors and customs that rise above borders.

1. Unique Event Recipes and Dinner Thoughts

Enjoy your faculties with an organized assortment of unique event recipes that catch the embodiment of Mediterranean celebrations. From delicious sheep sticks prepared with fragrant spices to tempting fish paella injected with saffron, each dish recounts an account of custom and festivity. Investigate the craft of meze, where little plates of olives, cheeses, and simmered vegetables meet up to make an ensemble of flavors, ideal for sharing and enjoying.

Plunge into the universe of Mediterranean desserts, where baklava's flaky layers and sweet nuts dance on the sense of taste. Find the mysteries of making the ideal couscous dish, a staple in Mediterranean eats that represents solidarity and overflow. These recipes tempt taste buds as well as act as an association with the district's rich social embroidery.

2. Empowering a Comprehensive Way to Deal with Prosperity

Past the extravagant banquets, Part 8 urges a comprehensive way to deal with prosperity, perceiving that genuine festival includes the body as well as the brain and soul. Dig into the Mediterranean way of life, where feasts are relished gradually, cultivating a feeling of care and appreciation.

Investigate the medical advantages of the Mediterranean eating regimen, eminent for its accentuation on new natural products, vegetables, entire grains, and olive oil. Find how these fixings make heavenly dishes as well as add to life span and prosperity. The Mediterranean way of life reaches out past the plate, incorporating an adoration for open-air exercises, social associations, and a profound appreciation for life's straightforward joys.

3. Culinary Practices for Foodies and Social Pioneers

Drench yourself in the dynamic embroidered artwork of culinary customs that characterize Mediterranean festivals. From the exuberant business sectors of Marrakech to the waterfront kitchens of Greece, this part welcomes foodies and social travelers to set out on a tactile experience.

Uncover the mysteries of safeguarding lemons in Morocco or become familiar with the specialty of creating the ideal Spanish paella in Valencia. Draw in with local people, share stories, and take part in respected customs that have been gone down through ages. Part 8 celebrates the demonstration of eating as well as the social accounts woven into each dish.

All in all, Part 8 is a festival of life, love, and the lively embroidery of Mediterranean occasions. Through exceptional event recipes, dinner thoughts, and a comprehensive way to deal with prosperity and culinary practices, it coaxes you to relish the experience, interface with others, and embrace the glad soul of the Mediterranean way of life. Enjoy the gala, sustain your spirit, and let the festival start.

CONCLUSION

As we finish up our groundbreaking process through Mediterranean feasting, it's fundamental to think about the rich embroidered artwork of flavors, culture, and essentialness that has woven together this culinary experience. The Mediterranean eating routine, famous for its medical advantages and delightful taste, has taken us on a gastronomic journey that rises above simple food.

In recapping this culinary campaign, we end up drenched in the fragrant scenes of olive forests, the zing of citrus organic products, and the flavorful notes of spices like oregano and rosemary. Each dish has been an ensemble of healthy fixings, a demonstration of the locale's obligation to sustain both body and soul.

Our investigation through this cookbook has not simply been a culinary visit; it's an encouragement to embrace essentialness and joy. Past the recipes lie the key to an even life, where the delight of getting ready and sharing a feast turns into a festival of good well-being and association. As we turn the pages, let us enjoy the flavors as well as assimilate the significant insight implanted in the Mediterranean way of life.

This culinary work of art stretches out a warm hug to a different interest group, perceiving the exceptional necessities of people with changing preferences, inclinations, and dietary prerequisites. Whether you're a carefully prepared gourmet specialist, a well-being cognizant devotee, or a fledgling in the kitchen, there's a spot for you inside these pages. The cookbook fills in as a compass, directing every peruser toward a customized excursion of culinary disclosure.

Recognizing the different embroidery of our crowd, we've created recipes that take care of a range of dietary decisions — from vegan enjoyments to delicious fish dishes. We comprehend that each peruser offers their own social impacts and culinary practices of real value, and this cookbook is a festival of that variety.

As we close this section, let the pages of this cookbook be something other than recipes; let them be a wellspring of motivation for a way of life that champions prosperity, satisfaction, and inclusivity. In embracing the Mediterranean soul, we leave on an excursion where the kitchen changes into a safe haven of wellbeing, satisfaction, and the common human experience through the affection for great food.